EMT
IIII➤FLASH REVIEW

EMT
||||FLASH REVIEW

2nd Edition

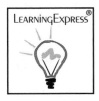

NEW YORK

Library of Congress Cataloging-in-Publication Data: on file

ISBN: 978-1-61103-050-1

Printed in the United States of America
9 8 7 6 5 4 3 2 1

For more information or to place an order, contact LearningExpress at:
    80 Broad Street
    Suite 400
    New York, NY 10004

ABOUT THE CONTRIBUTORS

Mike Clumpner is the founder and co-owner of NIMSHI International, based in Charlotte, North Carolina. NIMSHI specializes in providing training and consulting in the fields of homeland security, public safety, disaster response, tactical medicine, critical care medical education, and healthcare. Clumpner is also a full-time fire captain and paramedic for the Charlotte Fire Department, where he is assigned to the Special Operations Division. Clumpner spent five years as a tactical instructor for the United States Department of Justice, where he was responsible for creating training modules and instructing at the FBI Academy and the DEA Training Academy at their shared facilities in Quantico, Virginia.

He has undergraduate degrees in fire science, paramedicine, and business administration and a Master's degree in business administration, and is completing a doctoral degree in homeland security policy. Clumpner has also published numerous magazine articles and books on critical care medicine and homeland security and is a frequent lecturer on critical care medicine, public safety operations, and homeland security issues. He has lectured extensively throughout North America, South America, Central America, Europe, Australia, New Zealand, and the Caribbean, and has presented at over 170 congresses and symposiums.

Gregory R. Sharpe, MPA, is a battalion chief with the Charlotte Fire Department of Charlotte, North Carolina. He has been with the fire department for 18 years and has been a paramedic for 17 of those years. He began his EMS career as a volunteer for the

St. Michael's College Fire and Rescue Department in February of 1986. Sharpe has served for various law enforcement agencies as a law enforcement officer and for Mecklenburg EMS Agency as a paramedic crew chief, and has been an EMS instructor for the past 14 years. He earned his Master of Public Administration from the University of North Carolina at Charlotte in December 2009.

CONTENTS

HOW TO USE THIS BOOK

The flashcards in this book contain more than 650 terms that are commonly found on most EMS exams, and are also helpful for practicing EMTs who are looking to keep their skills sharp.

This book is organized into the six categories of the NREMT cognitive exam to help you study. The cognitive exam is broken down into the six categories, and your score will be broken down similarly. If you are having trouble in a specific area, you can focus your studying there. If you are trying to improve or keep your skills sharp, you can work your way through the different categories and focus on your weakest areas.

Note: As anatomy and physiology cross all categories, these terms are placed in the category where they are most likely to be encountered: the musculoskeletal and integumentary systems are under Trauma; the respiratory system, except airway anatomy (Airway), is under Respiration and Ventilation; the cardiovascular system is under Cardiology and Resuscitation; all other systems are under Medical/Obstetrics/Gynecology; and medical terminology and pharmacology are listed under EMS Operations.

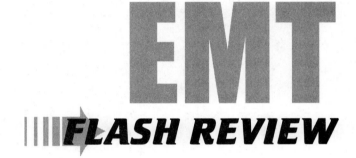

blind insertion airway device (BIAD)

carina

complete airway obstruction

AIRWAY

- an airway that is intended to occlude the esophagus to prevent aspiration and gastric distention, and to allow adequate artificial ventilations; examples of a BIAD are the King Airway, Combitube, and Laryngeal Mask Airway (LMA)

- the point in the lower end of the trachea where the two bronchi branch

- blockage of the airway from a foreign body or swelling of the tissues; the most common obstruction is the patient's own tongue, and a complete blockage is signified by the patient's inability to speak or with inadequate ventilator effort; see Appendix A for the procedures to relieve an airway obstruction

cricoid cartilage

cricothyroid membrane

cricothyrotomy

AIRWAY

- the only complete ring of cartilage in the trachea, located immediately below the larynx; the Sellick's maneuver may be performed here

- the membrane between the thyroid cartilage and the cricoid cartilage where emergency and surgical airways are performed

- an emergency airway established by puncturing the cricothyroid membrane

endotracheal tube

epiglottis

epiglottitis

AIRWAY

- a tube placed in the trachea to more effectively ventilate a patient and protect the lungs from aspiration

- the flap of tissue above the larynx that closes off the airway when a person swallows

- inflammation and swelling of the epiglottis, usually by bacterial infection, and potentially life threatening due to airway obstruction

AIRWAY

gag reflex

glottis

head-tilt, chin-lift maneuver

AIRWAY

- a reflex causing one to retch or make an effort to vomit

- opening between the vocal cords into the trachea

- a method of opening the airway, used when a patient is free from neck or spinal injury

Heimlich maneuver

intubation

jaw-thrust maneuver

AIRWAY

- a procedure consisting of a series of thrusts to the abdomen, designed to rid the airway of obstructions

- insertion of a tube; frequently the placement of an endotracheal tube into the trachea

- a method of opening the airway that avoids moving or extending the neck, often used in cases of trauma

laryngectomee

laryngectomy

laryngoscope

AIRWAY

- a patient who has had all or part of the larynx surgically removed

- the removal of the larynx, usually due to cancer of the larynx

- an instrument used to view the larynx, usually for the purpose of placing an endotracheal tube or removing a foreign body airway obstruction

laryngospasm

larynx

nasogastric tube

AIRWAY

- severe constriction or narrowing of the larynx, often due to an allergic reaction

- the voice box

- a tube that is inserted into the nose while the patient swallows, and goes into the stomach to facilitate drainage and/or feeding

nasopharyngeal airway

nasopharynx

oropharyngeal airway

AIRWAY

- a flexible plastic tube that is inserted into the nasal passageway to allow air to flow unobstructed

- back of the throat and nose

- a plastic device inserted into the mouth and posterior pharynx of an unresponsive patient without a gag reflex, used to keep the tongue from occluding the airway

oropharynx

partial airway obstruction

patent

AIRWAY

- area behind the base of the tongue and back of the mouth

- an incomplete blockage of the airway by a foreign body or swelling of the tissues; signs may include stridor or a hoarse cough; the patient should be encouraged to cough and supported with O_2 if it does not interfere with the patient clearing his or her own airway

- open; unobstructed

pharynx

rapid sequence intubation (RSI)

sniffing position

AIRWAY

- the throat

- orotracheal intubation, performed after temporarily
  sedating a patient with drugs

- placement of a child's head for endotracheal intubation

stoma

stridor

trachea

AIRWAY

- a small, artificial bodily opening usually made during surgery, such as a tracheostomy

- a high-pitched upper airway sound caused by the narrowing of the trachea or larynx

- the windpipe

tracheostomy

AIRWAY

- a surgical opening into the neck and trachea

accessory muscles of respiration

agonal

alveoli

- muscles that aid the diaphragm in breathing, especially when breathing is difficult, including intercostal muscles, abdominal muscles, and neck muscles

- respirations that are gasping, infrequent, and irregular, which are typical of a sick or dying patient

- the air sacs of the lungs, where oxygen and carbon dioxide exchange occurs

anoxia

apnea

artificial ventilation

RESPIRATION AND VENTILATION

- absence of oxygen

- the absence of breathing

- breathing for someone else by forcing air into his or her lungs

aspiration

asthma

bag valve mask (BVM)

RESPIRATION AND VENTILATION

- inhaling a foreign substance, such as food or vomitus, into the airway or lungs

- a respiratory disorder in which there is a spasm of the small air passages and mucus production occurs, resulting in labored breathing and wheezing

- a device used to provide artificial ventilation

beta-2 receptor

beta agonist bronchodilator

blow-by oxygen delivery

RESPIRATION AND VENTILATION

- located in the lungs and when stimulated by epinephrine causes the bronchioles to dilate

- a common, inhaled medication used for shortness of breath and dilating the bronchi by relaxing the muscles surrounding the bronchioles

- oxygen delivery method for infants, performed by holding an oxygen mask close to the infant's mouth and nose

bronchi

bronchioles

bronchitis

- the two main airway tubes, which come off the trachea and go to the lungs

- airway branches that carry air to and from the air sacs (alveoli)

- a chronic obstructive pulmonary disease (COPD) that includes inflammation and irritation of the bronchi and bronchioles

bronchoconstriction

bronchodilator

capnograph

RESPIRATION AND VENTILATION

- narrowing or constricting of the bronchi and bronchioles

- a medication that opens the airways to ease breathing difficulty

- instrument used to measure concentration of exhaled carbon dioxide in an air sample

carbon dioxide (CO_2)

Cheyne-Stokes respiration

chronic obstructive pulmonary disease (COPD or COLD)

RESPIRATION AND VENTILATION

- a gas formed by respiration in the body and exhaled

- an abnormal breathing pattern signified by alternating between an increasing rate and depth and periods of apnea

- a disease of the respiratory system, commonly chronic bronchitis or emphysema, that results in narrowed airways

crackles

croup

cyanosis

RESPIRATION AND VENTILATION

- low-pitched, abnormal lung sounds caused by fluid in the smaller airways; sometimes called rhonchi

- a common viral respiratory tract infection in infants and children, characterized by spasms of the larynx and/or a barking cough

- a bluish or gray coloring of the mucous membranes and skin, usually around the mouth, fingertips, or earlobes, which indicates severe lack of oxygenation to body tissue

demand valve

dyspnea

emphysema

RESPIRATION AND VENTILATION

- also known as a flow-restricted, oxygen-powered ventilation device (FROPVD) or manually triggered ventilation device (MTVD); a device that delivers oxygen under high pressures and can be operated by one EMT with a two-handed mask seal

- difficult, labored breathing

- a chronic obstructive pulmonary disease (COPD) resulting in the loss of elasticity of the lungs

exhalation

FiO$_2$ (fraction of inspired oxygen)

flowmeter

RESPIRATION AND VENTILATION

- to breathe air out of the lungs

- oxygen concentration of inspired air, measured in percentage, with Fi02 of 1.0 equaling 100 percent concentration of oxygen

- a device connected to an oxygen cylinder that measures the amount of oxygen being delivered

hemoglobin

humidifier

hyperventilation

- the oxygen-carrying pigment of red blood cells

- a device that uses water to provide moisture to the oxygen coming from an oxygen delivery system

- increased rate and/or depth of respiration

hypoventilation

hypoxemia

hypoxia

RESPIRATION AND VENTILATION

- inadequate ventilation rate or volume to sustain oxygenation

- inadequate oxygen in the blood

- inadequate oxygen in the blood being delivered to body tissue

inhalation

inhaler

inspiration

RESPIRATION AND VENTILATION

- breathing in; drawing air into the lungs; also a rate of medication administration and exposure to toxins

- a device that provides an aerosol form of medication into the airway, usually a bronchodilator

- breathing in; drawing air into the lungs

lungs

nasal cannula

nebulizer

RESPIRATION AND VENTILATION

- organs in the thoracic cavity where the exchange of gas, primarily oxygen and carbon dioxide, occurs

- an oxygen delivery device, consisting of two prongs that go into the nose

- a device that delivers water or liquid medication in the form of a fine spray or mist

non-rebreather mask

orthopnea

oxygen

RESPIRATION AND VENTILATION

- an oxygen delivery device that contains a mask with a bag and delivers about 90 percent oxygen

- severe difficulty in breathing that occurs when lying down and is typically relieved by sitting up

- odorless, colorless gas that is essential to sustaining life; normal air contains 21 percent oxygen

paroxysmal nocturnal dyspnea

pH (potential of hydrogen)

pleura

RESPIRATION AND VENTILATION

- nighttime coughing or shortness of breath

- a scale representing the relative acidity or alkalinity of a substance; normal body pH range is 7.35 to 7.45

- the lining of the lungs, which consists of two layers; the visceral layer covers the lungs and the parietal layer lines the chest cavity

pleural space

pleuritis

pneum-

- the potential space between the pleura, which normally contains a small amount of fluid

- inflammation of the pleura

- a word root meaning *lung*

pneumonia

pneumothorax

Positive Pressure Ventilation (PPV)

RESPIRATION AND VENTILATION

- infection of the lungs

- a condition involving air in the pleural cavity due to injury or disease

  There are three types of pneumothoraxes: (1) spontaneous pneumothorax results from illness or genetic weakness in the lung wall and is most commonly seen in tall, thin individuals; (2) simple pneumothorax involves air in the pleural cavity without signs and symptoms of severe respiratory distress; (3) tension pneumothorax presents with severe respiratory distress and requires immediate surgical intervention for survival

- any of several techniques used to provide artificial ventilations by forcing air into the lungs; techniques include mouth-to-mask, bag-valve mask, and demand valve ventilations

RESPIRATION AND VENTILATION

pulmonary

pulmonary edema

pulse oximeter

RESPIRATION AND VENTILATION

- having to do with the lungs

- fluid in the lungs

- device that measures the percentage of bound hemoglobin in the blood

rales

rescue breathing

respiration

RESPIRATION AND VENTILATION

- lung crackles; abnormal breath sounds

- artificially breathing for a patient who has stopped breathing

- the exchange of oxygen and carbon dioxide at the alveolar level

respiratory arrest

respiratory distress

respiratory failure

RESPIRATION AND VENTILATION

- cessation of respiration/breathing

- difficulty breathing

- a state of inadequate oxygenation and/or ventilation

retractions

rhonchi

Sellick's maneuver

RESPIRATION AND VENTILATION

- a possible indication of respiratory distress, where the skin pulls tightly around the ribs, above the clavicles, or in the sternal notch during inspiration

- abnormally coarse, rattling breath sounds

- external pressure on the anterior cricoid cartilage, used to occlude the esophagus and prevent aspiration

tachypnea

thorax

tidal volume

RESPIRATION AND VENTILATION

- rapid respiratory rate

- the chest cavity, containing the heart and lungs

- the volume of inspired or expired air in a single breath

tuberculosis

ventilation

wheeze

- a chronic, contagious infection, usually affecting the lungs

- the provision of air to the lungs

- a high-pitched whistling noise indicating narrowed lower airways; asthma, COPD, or an allergic reaction may be the cause

acute myocardial infarction (AMI)

advanced cardiac life support (ACLS)

afterload

- death of a portion of the heart muscle due to lack of blood and oxygen; a heart attack

- fourth link in the chain of survival in cardiac care, including airway control and intravenous drugs, and consisting of: (1) early access; (2) early CPR; (3) early defibrillation; and (4) early advanced care

- the pressure against which the left ventricle must pump

alpha receptors

angina pectoris

antidysrhythmics

- sites in the blood vessels that cause constriction and an increase in blood pressure when stimulated by epinephrine

- pain, discomfort, or pressure localized in the chest caused by ischemia; it is categorized as stable (discomfort brought on by exertion and relieved by rest or low dose nitroglycerin) or unstable (discomfort that is different than other occurrences of angina, i.e., onset with less exertion or at rest and no relief with rest, or an increased dose of nitroglycerin required for relief)

- a category of drugs that manage and prevent electrocardiography rhythm disturbances

antihypertensive

aorta

arrhythmia

CARDIOLOGY AND RESUSCITATION

- a category of drugs that manages high blood pressure

- the largest artery in the body, which receives blood from the left ventricle and delivers it to arteries that supply the limbs and all organs except the lungs

- a disturbance in the heart rhythm or rate

arteriole

arteriosclerosis

artery

- the smallest kind of artery, which connects to the capillaries

- an arterial disorder that decreases the arteries' ability to effectively carry blood to the body

- a blood vessel that carries blood away from the heart

asystole

atherosclerosis

atrial fibrillation

- no electrical impulses from the heart, resulting in no pumping and a straight-line ECG reading

- a type of arterio sclerosis signified by a thickened, diseased condition of the arteries, due to cholesterol buildup, that prevents them from efficiently carrying blood

- an ECG rhythm where a pacemaker is in the atria and electrical activity there is chaotic, resulting in an irregular pulse

atrium

automated external defibrillator (AED)

automaticity

- one of the two upper chambers of the heart (right or left)

- a portable device that identifies either ventricular tachycardia (V-Tach) or ventricular fibrillation (V-Fib) and either automatically delivers a shock (AED) or advises the user that a shock should be delivered (semi-automated external defibrillator, or SAED)

- the unique ability of cardiac pacemaker cells to initiate an impulse without an external stimulus

baroreceptor

beta blocker

beta-1 receptor

CARDIOLOGY AND RESUSCITATION

- a sensing mechanism in the aortic arch and carotid sinus that detects changes in pressure in the vascular system

- a drug that antagonizes action of the adrenergic receptors of the sympathetic nervous system, resulting in decreased heart rate and dilation of cardiac vessels

- located in the heart and when stimulated by epinephrine causes an increase in rate and strength of contractility

brachial pulse

bradycardia

bruit

CARDIOLOGY AND RESUSCITATION

- the pulse point found on the inside of the upper arm; the most common site to check the pulse on an infant during CPR

- a slow heart rate—fewer than 60 beats per minute

- a sound emitted when blood meets a partial obstruction

cardiac arrest

cardiac compromise

cardiac output

CARDIOLOGY AND RESUSCITATION

- condition where the heart stops beating or pumping

- a term referring to a heart-related problem that results in inadequate perfusion to organs

- the amount of blood pumped by the heart in one minute; it is calculated by multiplying the stroke volume by the heart rate per minute

cardiac standstill

cardiopulmonary arrest

cardiopulmonary resuscitation (CPR)

CARDIOLOGY AND RESUSCITATION

- cardiac arrest; cessation of the heart

- cessation of cardiac contractions and spontaneous respirations

- basic life support procedures including call for help, initial assessment, opening the airway, artificial breathing, and manual external cardiac compressions

carotid pulse

carotid sinus massage

circulatory system

- the pulse point on each side of the neck, checked during adult and child CPR

- use of pressure on the carotid sinus, in the carotid artery, to convert certain abnormal heart rhythms to a normal rhythm

- the heart, blood, and blood vessels

congestive heart failure (CHF)

cor pulmonale

coronary arteries

- failure of the heart to effectively pump, causing backup of blood and fluid into the lungs (left-sided failure) and/or the body (right-sided failure)

- an enlarging (hypertrophy) of the right ventricle usually secondary to lung disease; it may lead to congestive heart failure

- the blood vessels that supply blood to the heart muscle

CARDIOLOGY AND RESUSCITATION

coronary artery disease

defibrillation

diastole

- the narrowing of the coronary arteries in one or more places, which can lead to complete blockage and damage to the heart muscle

- electrical shock delivered to a patient's heart to correct ventricular fibrillation or ventricular tachycardia without a pulse

- period of ventricular relaxation in which the ventricles fill with blood

diastolic (blood) pressure

diuretic

dysrhythmia

- arterial pressure when the heart is relaxed

- water pill; a medication used to increase excretion of water from the body, typically for treatment of congestive heart failure

- abnormal electrical activity in the heart

electrocardiogram (ECG)

electrode

electrolyte

- a graphic representation of the electrical activity of the heart, produced by the depolarization and repolarization of the atria and ventricles

- a wire or patch that connects the patient to an electrocardiogram (ECG) machine and measures the electrical activity of the heart

- a substance that, when put in water, separates into particles that can conduct an electric current

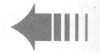

embolus

embolism

endocarditis

- something that travels through the bloodstream and can get stuck, such as a blood clot, fat particle, or air bubble

- occlusion due to movement of a blood clot, fat particle, or air bubble in a blood vessel from another part of the body·

- inflammation of the inside lining of the heart

endocardium

erythrocyte

femoral pulse

CARDIOLOGY AND RESUSCITATION

- the thin inside lining or membrane of the heart

- red blood cell

- the pulse point in the groin

fibrillation

heart attack

hypertension

CARDIOLOGY AND RESUSCITATION

- chaotic, unorganized electrical activity of the heart, which results in irregular pumping; can involve the atria, ventricles, or both

- a nonmedical term for an acute myocardial infarction; heart-muscle damage due to lack of blood flow

- high blood pressure

hypertrophy

infarction

ischemia

- an increase in the size of body tissue or an organ due to an increase in the size of the cells

- necrosis; tissue death due to lack of blood supply

- lack of blood flow to tissue, usually from severe narrowing of an artery or an obstruction

leukocyte

mediastinum

myocardial infarction

- a white blood cell

- the area separating the left and right lungs, which contains the heart, great vessels (aorta, superior vena cava, inferior vena cava), esophagus, and trachea

- heart attack; death of a portion of the heart muscle due to an inadequate amount of blood supply

myocardium

normal sinus rhythm (NSR)

occlusion

- the heart muscle

- the normal rhythm of the heart, where an electrical impulse arises from the sinoatrial node and travels through the heart's normal pathways without interference

- a blockage, usually referring to a blocked blood vessel

palpitation

pericarditis

pericardium

CARDIOLOGY AND RESUSCITATION

- a sensation of heart fluttering or irregularity caused by dysrhythmia

- inflammation of the pericardium

- the membrane around the heart

plasma

preload

pulmonary artery

- the fluid component of blood

- the amount of blood returning to the ventricle

- the major artery coming from the right ventricle of the heart, which carries nonoxygenated blood to the lungs

pulmonary veins

radial pulse

serum

CARDIOLOGY AND RESUSCITATION

- the major veins coming from the lungs, which carry oxygenated blood to the left atrium of the heart

- the pulse point on the wrist, most often used when determining an individual's pulse rate

- liquid portion of blood remaining after coagulation

stenosis

synchronized cardioversion

systole

- narrowing of a body orifice or passageway

- an electrical shock through the heart, at a specific time during the cardiac cycle, intended to terminate dysrhythmia

- contraction of the heart

systolic pressure

tachycardia

thrombus

CARDIOLOGY AND RESUSCITATION

- arterial pressure when the heart is contracting

- rapid heart beat, usually over 100 beats per minute

- a blood clot

vascular

vasoconstriction

vasodilation

- pertaining to blood vessels

- narrowing of the lumen or diameter of blood vessels

- widening of the lumen or diameter of blood vessels

vena cava

ventricles

ventricular fibrillation (VF)

- a major vein of the body that returns blood to the right side of the heart; the inferior vena cava delivers blood from areas below the heart and the superior vena cava delivers blood from areas above the heart

- can be found in both the heart (the two lower chambers) and the brain (small cavities that produce and store cerebral spinal fluid)

- an ECG rhythm characterized by chaotic electrical impulses in the ventricle; this rhythm does not result in pumping and requires immediate defibrillation

ventricular tachycardia

- a life-threatening rapid ECG rhythm with the ventricle as an abnormal pacemaker; this rhythm may or may not produce mechanical pumping

abrasion

amputation

angulated

TRAUMA

- a scrape or scratch of the skin

- the complete removal of a limb or part of the body

- deformed; at an angle

arachnoid membrane

arterial gas embolism (AGE)

avulsion

TRAUMA

- the middle of the three layers of the meninges, named after its spiderlike structure

- blockage of blood vessels by air bubbles; usually encountered during dive emergencies; symptoms vary as to the location of the embolism, with one of the most serious being a cerebral arterial gas embolism (CAGE)

- an open soft tissue injury with a flap of tissue remaining or the tissue completely torn off

bandage

barotrauma

Battle's sign

TRAUMA

- a material used to keep a dressing on a wound in place

- injury from increased pressure inside the body's air-filled cavities, which often occurs during diving descent; the most common barotrauma is a ruptured eardrum

- bruising behind the ears, which usually indicates a fracture at the base of the skull

Beck's triad

bends

capillary refill

TRAUMA

- three classic characteristics of cardiac tamponade: muffled heart sounds, narrowing pulse pressure, and neck vein distention

- a condition caused by bubbles of nitrogen gas in the blood, which occurs during a rapid ascent from deepwater diving; a common symptom of decompression sickness

- a test to evaluate for hypoperfusion in an infant or child, wherein the examiner presses firmly on the patient's skin to blanch (whiten) the area and measures the time it takes for skin to pink up

cardiac tamponade

cervical collar

clavicle

TRAUMA

- a condition whereby cardiac contraction is greatly reduced due to blood or fluid in the pericardial sac; also called pericardial tamponade

- a rigid brace used to stabilize and minimize neck movement after injury

- collar bone

closed fracture

closed head injury

coccyx

TRAUMA

- a break in a bone that does not open the skin

- head trauma that results in swelling and/or bleeding within the skull without an opening to the environment

- tail bone; the last four bones of the spinal column, which are fused together

concussion

crepitus

Cushing's triad

TRAUMA

- a minor head injury, usually accompanied by transient loss of consciousness

- the sound of broken bone ends rubbing together

- signs often observed in patients with increased intracranial pressure, including decreased pulse rate, increased blood pressure, and changes in respiration

decerebrate posturing

decompression sickness

decorticate posturing

- the posture of an unconscious patient, in which the arms and legs are extended; this usually indicates severe intracranial pressure on the brain stem

- an injury that occurs from ascending from a dive too quickly, not performing a safety stop, or remaining at depth for too long, resulting in bubbles (usually nitrogen) being trapped in tissues or blood vessels, with symptom onset as late as 72 hours post-dive

- the posture of an unconscious patient, in which the arms are flexed and the legs are extended or possibly flexed; often indicates increased intracranial pressure and significant brain injury

deformity

dermis

direct pressure

TRAUMA

- an abnormal shape

- the second layer of the skin, found right below the epidermis

- a method of stopping bleeding that involves putting a firm hold on the bleeding site

dislocation

dressing

drowning

TRAUMA

- disruption of a joint

- protective covering for a wound, to help stop bleeding and prevent contamination

- respiratory impairment due to submersion in liquid, regardless of the outcome

TRAUMA

ecchymosis

edema

epidermis

TRAUMA

- bruising

- swelling of body tissue due to excess fluid

- the outermost layer of skin

epidural hematoma

eschar

eviscerate

TRAUMA

- a condition in which blood accumulates in the epidural space

- the dry, stiff, necrotic tissue resulting from a burn

- to remove an organ from a patient; disembowel

exsanguinate

femur

fibula

TRAUMA

- the act of draining or losing blood

- thigh bone

- the small, outermost bone in the lower leg

flail chest

fracture

frontal

TRAUMA

- condition in which two or more ribs are broken in two or more places, creating an unstable chest wall that ineffectively supports ventilation

- a break in a bone or solid organ

- pertaining to the forehead

frostbite

full-thickness burn

Glasgow Coma Scale (GCS)

TRAUMA

- a cold injury where the tissue freezes and is damaged

- a third-degree burn, affecting all layers of skin

- a numeric scale reflecting a quick assessment of central nervous system function, including eye opening, verbal responsiveness, and motor responsiveness; see Appendix G

golden hour/period

guarding

heat cramps

TRAUMA

- a patient has the best chance for survival if he or she arrives in the operating room within 60 minutes of the traumatic injury

- when patients voluntarily tighten their abdominal muscles to protect their abdominal area because of pain or injury

- lower extremity and abdominal muscle cramping due to fluid and salt loss from heat exposure

heat exhaustion

heatstroke

hematoma

TRAUMA

- a condition of weakness and dizziness due to excessive fluid loss from heat exposure

- sunstroke; severe hyperthermia due to exposure to high environmental temperatures

- a collection of blood in body tissue, due to an injured blood vessel

hematuria

hemoptysis

hemorrhage

TRAUMA

- blood in the urine

- the coughing up of blood

- a rapid and uncontrollable loss of blood

hemothorax

hip

humerus

TRAUMA

- blood in the pleural space, between the lungs and the chest wall

- the joint at the top of the thigh, located between the thigh and the pelvis

- the bone of the upper arm

hyperextension

hyperthermia

hypoperfusion

TRAUMA

- the overextension of a limb

- having an extremely high body temperature

- a state of inadequate perfusion, or blood flow, to the body; shock

hypotension

hypothermia

hypovolemia

TRAUMA

- a condition of abnormally low blood pressure

- a condition of having an extremely low body temperature

- a disorder resulting in low or inadequate volume of blood in the circulatory system

hypovolemic shock

immobilize

integumentary system

TRAUMA

- hypoperfusion due to inadequate body fluid or blood

- to hold a part firmly in place; to restrict motion

- the body system consisting of the skin, hair, and nails

intercostal

joint

laceration

TRAUMA

- the space between the ribs

- place where two bones come together

- a tearing or cutting wound

ligaments

mandible

maxilla

TRAUMA

- fibrous connective tissue that joins and connects bones and strengthens joints

- the lower jawbone

- the immovable upper bone of the jaw

mechanism of injury

metacarpals

metatarsals

TRAUMA

- the cause and method of an injury; considerations include type, intensity, direction of force, and body parts affected

- the bones of the hand between the wrist and the fingers

- the bones of the foot between the ankle and the toes

midclavicular line

musculoskeletal system

occipital

TRAUMA

- an anatomical landmark consisting of an imaginary line from the middle of the clavicle downward to the chest

- the system of bones, joints, muscles, and related structures that enable the body to move and function

- the posterior area of the head including the base of the skull; the occipital bone is sutured to the two parietal and temporal bones

open head injury

parietal

partial-thickness burn

TRAUMA

- a head injury with an opening that could allow bacteria to enter

- the superior region of the head; here are two parietal bones sutured to each other and to the frontal, temporal, and occipital bones

- second-degree burn; a burn in which the top layer or epidermis is burned and some of the dermis is injured

pelvis

perfusion

pericardial tamponade

TRAUMA

- the bones of the lower trunk of the body

- providing oxygen and nutrients to the cells and removing wastes to meet the current cellular requirements

- a condition in which there is a dangerous excess of blood or fluid inside the pericardial sac

phalanges

pneumatic antishock garment (PASG)

position of function

- finger or toe bones

- MAST (military anti-shock trousers); inflatable trouser-like garment that may be effective in managing shock and stabilizing pelvic fractures

- natural, relaxed body positions that preserve normal function

pressure dressing

pressure point

priapism

- bulky, tightly secured bandages that provide direct pressure and help control bleeding

- the site of a major artery close to the surface of the body, where it was once believed direct pressure could stop bleeding distal to the site; this is no longer an accepted practice

- sustained penile erection, sometimes due to a spinal cord injury or other medical condition

pulse pressure

raccoon eyes

radius

TRAUMA

- the difference between the systolic and diastolic pressure; a narrowing of the pulse pressure may indicate a cardiac tamponade

- bruising around the eye area, usually indicating a fracture in the base of the skull

- the bone of the forearm, on the thumb side

Revised Trauma Score (RTS)

rule of nines

scapula

TRAUMA

- a scoring system to gauge the severity of a patient's injuries; it uses the Glasgow Coma Scale (GCS), systolic blood pressure, and respiratory rate to predict survival probabilities; as the score decreases, the probability the patient survives also decreases; most common scoring system for patients with head injuries; see appendix H

- a method of estimating the total percentage of burned body surface area, using the principle that the adult human body can be divided into anatomic regions with surface areas that are multiples of nine percent

- shoulder blade

shock

skull

sling

TRAUMA

- 1. inadequate perfusion resulting in rapid disruption in one's physical and mental faculties, which often follows serious injury; 2. discharge of electrical energy, as in defibrillation

- the bony structure of the head made up of two sets of bones: (1) the cranium, made up of four sutured bones: the frontal (forehead); two temporal bones (temples); parietal (top); and occiput (rear/base); and (2) the facial bones, made up of the nasal, zygomatic, maxillae (immovable), and mandible (movable) bones

- a bandage applied around the neck to support and immobilize the lower arm

sprain

sternum

strain

TRAUMA

- a ligament injury, either by abnormal stretching or partial tear

- the breast bone

- a minor muscle injury due to overexertion

TRAUMA

subdural hematoma

swathe

temporal

TRAUMA

- accumulation of blood between the pia mater and the arachnoid membrane

- a band tied around a portion of the body, used to aid immobilization

- the area of the head around the temples and ears; there are two temporal bones that are sutured to the parietal and occipital bones

tendon

thoracotomy

tibia

TRAUMA

- connective tissue that joins muscle to bone

- surgical opening of the chest

- the shinbone or medial lower leg bone

tourniquet

traction splint

trauma

TRAUMA

- used if direct pressure fails to control bleeding; may be commercially made or improvised with a wide cloth and windlass

- fracture stabilization device that exerts force to straighten and align the bone ends of a femur fracture

- injury by an external force; usually a physical injury, but can be psychological

traumatic asphyxia

tympanic membrane

ulna

TRAUMA

- a severe, life-threatening injury to the chest that forces blood from the heart to the upper chest, neck, and face

- the eardrum

- the larger bone of the forearm on the little finger side

vertebrae

vertebral

xiphoid process

TRAUMA

- the individual bones of the spinal cord

- pertaining to the spinal column

- the cartilage at the lower tip of the sternum

zygoma

TRAUMA

- the cheekbone in the human skull

abortion

abruptio placentae

acclimatization

- miscarriage; termination of pregnancy, either spontaneously or as a result of inducement

- premature separation of the placenta from the uterine wall, which can be partial or complete, and usually painful

- the body's physical adaptation to a different climate or elevation

acquired immune deficiency syndrome (AIDS)

activated charcoal

acute glaucoma

- an advanced stage of the human immunodeficiency virus infection, during which the body's immune system is severely compromised

- a powder, usually premixed with water, that adsorbs various toxic ingestions in the stomach and prevents absorption in the body

- acute increase in eye pressure, which can cause permanent blindness if left untreated

alkalosis

allergen

allergic reaction

- a body pH above 7.45, indicating a low concentration of hydrogen ions

- an external agent, such as an insect sting, food, or medication, that causes an allergic reaction

- a hypersensitive reaction to an allergen, typically characterized by itching, skin rash, swelling, wheezing, and hypoperfusion

Alzheimer's disease

amniotic fluid

amphetamines

- a type of dementia that leads to a progressive loss of mental ability and deterioration of memory

- the fluid that surrounds a baby in the amniotic sac prior to birth

- the central nervous system (CNS) stimulant category of drugs that typically causes general mood elevation

anaphylaxis; anaphylactic shock

anemia

aneurysm

- an often severe, life-threatening allergic reaction that typically leads to hypoperfusion and respiratory distress

- a low amount of red blood cells in the blood

- a ballooning or dilation of a weakened blood vessel, usually an artery, due to atherosclerosis, hypertension, infection, or trauma

antagonist

anticoagulant

antidote

MEDICAL / OBSTETRICS / GYNECOLOGY

- a drug that blocks the action of another drug's action

- a drug that inhibits clotting

- a substance that will counteract or neutralize the effects of a poison

antiemetic

antitussive

APGAR

- a category of drugs that reduce or eliminate nausea and vomiting

- a category of drugs that suppress the cough reflex

- a standardized assessment for newborns taken at one minute and five minutes after birth; the areas of assessment are **A**ppearance, **P**ulse, **G**rimace or irritability, **A**ctivity or muscle tone, and **R**espiration

autoimmunity

autonomic nervous system (ANS)

bag of waters

- a pathological condition whereby an individual has an immune response to his or her own tissues

- the portion of the nervous system that controls involuntary functions such as cardiac muscle and glands. The sympathetic nervous system and the parasympathetic nervous system are the two divisions.

- the sac of amniotic fluid that surrounds a baby in the uterus

barbiturates

benzodiazepines

bile

- a category of drugs that depress the central nervous system and cause sleep

- a category of drugs that decrease anxiety and lead to sedation

- fluid secreted by the liver and stored in the gallbladder that helps digest fats

biotransformation

bipolar disorder

bloody show

- the chemical modification of a substance within the body

- periods of excessive excitement and depression

- mucous and blood discharge from the vagina; a signal of impending labor

brain stem

breech presentation

buccal

- the lower portion of the brain, which is continuous with the spinal cord

- event in which a baby's buttocks or legs appear first during birth

- related to, near, or involving the cheek

capillary

carbon monoxide (CO)

central nervous system (CNS)

- the smallest blood vessels, where gases (primarily oxygen and carbon dioxide) are exchanged

- a colorless, odorless, and poisonous gas created during combustion

- body system that includes the brain and spinal cord

cephalic presentation

cerebrospinal fluid (CSF)

cerebrovascular accident (CVA)

- the delivery position where the baby's head appears first during birth; also called vertex position

- the clear and watery fluid that surrounds the brain and spinal cord

- a stroke; the lack of blood to a region of the brain caused by thrombus, embolism, or hemorrhage

chemoreceptor

cholinergic

chronic

- a nerve cell that is sensitive to stimulation by chemical substances

- effects from the parasympathetic nervous system related to the neurotransmitter acetylcholine

- of long duration

colitis

colloid

colostomy

- inflammation of the colon

- intravenous solution that contains large molecules, such as proteins and starches, that cannot pass through capillary membranes and thus remain in the vascular system

- a surgical opening between the colon and the surface of the abdomen, used to drain colon contents

coma

comatose

constrict

- a state of total mental and physical unresponsiveness

- in a coma

- to become smaller and/or narrower

crowning

crystalloids

dehydration

- when part of a baby's head is seen through the vaginal opening during delivery

- intravenous fluids, such as five percent dextrose in water (D5W), normal saline, or Ringer's lactate, that do not contain protein or other large molecules

- excessive loss of body water or salt

delirium

delirium tremens (DTs)

delusion

- an acute state of confusion

- the most severe complications of alcohol withdrawal; symptoms include restlessness, agitation, hallucinations, trembling hands, and possibly seizures

- a false belief

dementia

diabetes

diabetic coma

- mental confusion and deterioration over a period of time

- a deficiency or absence of insulin production by the pancreas, rendering the body unable to use sugar

- severe diabetic ketoacidosis; severe hyperglycemia due to inadequate insulin production

diabetic ketoacidosis

diaphoresis

diaphragm

- severe diabetic ketoacidosis; severe hyperglycemia due to inadequate insulin production

- hyperglycemia with acidosis and the production of ketones

- the major muscle involved in respiration; separates the chest from the abdomen

dilate

diplopia

disorientation

- to open, enlarge, or expand in diameter

- double vision

- unable to discern one's name, location, time, or current circumstances

distal

distended

diverticula

- an anatomical term describing a position near the end of an extremity or farther away from the body; opposite of proximal

- swollen and/or stretched

- pockets of weakened tissue in the colon wall

diverticulitis

dorsal

dorsalis pedis (pedal pulse)

- inflammation of diverticula

- an anatomical term referring to the back or posterior side of the body

- a pulse in the top of the foot

downer

dura mater

dysfunction

- a slang expression for a medication that depresses the central nervous system and causes relaxation

- the outermost and strongest layer of the meninges, the covering of the brain

- abnormal or disturbed functioning

dysmenorrhea

dysphagia

dysplasia

- painful menstruation

- difficult or painful swallowing

- abnormal changes in cells or cell development, sometimes indicating a precancerous state

dystonic reaction

dysuria

eclampsia

- muscle stiffness or contraction that may cause distortion and twisted movements, typically in facial or neck muscles, and related to ingestion of some categories of medications

- painful or difficult urinating

- a severe complication of pregnancy, characterized by seizures and preceded by headaches, swelling (edema), and high blood pressure

ectopic pregnancy

effacement

efficacy

- an abnormal pregnancy that occurs when an egg is implanted outside the uterus

- the thinning of the cervix in preparation for delivery

- a drug's ability to produce an expected and intended result

effusion

emesis

encephalitis

- fluid leakage into a cavity, such as a joint or pleural space

- the act of vomiting

- inflammation of the brain

endocrine system

enteritis

enzyme

MEDICAL / OBSTETRICS / GYNECOLOGY

- the body system that includes the glands and produces hormones

- inflammation of the small intestine

- a protein that stimulates and hastens a chemical reaction

epidural space

epilepsy

epinephrine (adrenaline)

- the outermost part of the spinal canal; the potential space between the dura mater and the skull

- a general term for a seizure disorder that includes abnormal focus of electrical activity in the brain

- a naturally occurring catecholamine hormone secreted by the adrenal medulla; it can increase blood pressure, stimulate the heart muscle, accelerate the heart rate, and increase cardiac output, and is used for cardiac emergencies, severe allergic reactions, and as a bronchodilator

epistaxis

esophagus

etiology

- nosebleed

- the muscular tube that carries swallowed food from the throat to the stomach

- cause of a disease or condition; the study of causes of diseases

exacerbation

expectorant

extravasation

- the worsening of a disease or condition

- a medication to loosen up bronchial secretions and facilitate the ability to cough

- the leakage of fluids out of blood vessels and into the surrounding tissue

extremities

exudate

fainting

- the arms and legs

- pus or serum

- loss of consciousness, typically due to lack of blood to the brain; also called syncope

fallopian tubes

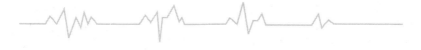

febrile

feces

- the structures that carry eggs from the ovaries to the uterus

- feverish

- bowel movement; evacuated waste from the intestines

fetus

flaccid

fontanels

- unborn child

- weak, flabby, lacking muscle tone

- the soft spots in the skulls of infants; openings in the skull prior to bone fusion

fundus (uterine)

gallbladder

gangrene

- the rounded or top part of the uterus

- an organ in the digestive system that stores bile and is located adjacent to the liver

- soft tissue death due to lack of blood supply

gastrointestinal

genitalia

genitourinary system

- related to the stomach and intestines

- the organs of the male and female reproductive systems

- the body system that includes the reproductive and urine-producing organs

gestation

glaucoma

glucose

- the period from conception to birth

- abnormally high pressure in an eye, leading to pain, redness, and vision loss

- sugar used by the body and metabolized to create energy

grand mal seizure

gravid

gravidity

- a generalized seizure with periods of intense involuntary muscle contractions and unconsciousness

- pregnant

- an individual's total number of pregnancies, including miscarriages

hallucination

hallucinogens

hematemesis

- experiencing a sensation (visual, auditory, tactile) that does not exist in reality

- a group of mind-altering drugs that create hallucinations or distort reality

- the vomiting of blood

hematocrit

hemiparesis

hemiplegia

- the percentage of red blood cells in a sample of whole blood; normal value is from 40 to 50 percent, depending on gender

- weakness on one side of the body

- paralysis of a vertical half of the body

hemodialysis

hemolysis

hemophilia

- the filtering or removal of waste products from the blood, which becomes necessary when the kidneys fail

- the breakdown or destruction of red blood cells

- an inherited blood clotting disorder

hemostasis

hepatitis

herniation

- the stopping of bleeding

- inflammation of the liver, due to either a virus or a toxic chemical

- the protrusion of an organ through an abnormal opening

hives

homeostasis

hormone

- a skin disorder usually associated with allergic reactions and characterized by redness, swelling, and itching; also called urticaria

- the appropriate balance or stability within the body

- a substance created in one part of the body that stimulates or regulates activity in another part

huffing

human immunodeficiency virus (HIV)

hyperglycemia

- street slang referring to illicit or illegal inhalation of chemicals

- the virus that causes acquired immune deficiency syndrome (AIDS)

- having a high blood sugar level

hypersensitivity

hypoglycemia

hypothalamus

- an abnormal susceptibility or allergy to a specific agent

- a condition of abnormally decreased blood sugar, usually anything less than 60 mg/dl

- the portion of the brain that regulates temperature, sleep, appetite, and other body functions

idiopathic

immune system

incontinence

- having an unknown origin or cause

- the body's defense system, which fights disease and foreign bodies; comprises white blood cells, the lymphatic system, antibodies, and body functions

- inability to control elimination of urine or feces

infection

insulin

insulin shock

- invasion of the body by a pathological microorganism, such as a bacteria or virus

- hormone secreted by the pancreas that allows the body to use sugar

- severe hypoglycemia; low blood sugar that may be characterized by abnormal behavior, a decreased level of consciousness, and seizures

islets of Langerhans

jaundice

jugular venous distention (JVD)

- lies within the pancreas and produces the hormones insulin, which decreases blood sugar levels in the blood, and glucagon, which increases blood sugar levels in the blood

- a yellowish coloration of the skin or eyes due to excessive bile pigments in the blood; usually a sign of liver disease

- bulging or distention of the jugular neck veins

ketoacidosis

kidneys

Kussmaul respirations

- a hyperglycemic condition in which acids and ketones are produced that may occur in diabetics

- paired organs that filter waste material from the blood

- respiratory pattern characteristic of diabetic patients in ketoacidosis, resulting in rapid and deep respirations

labor

lactation

lesion

- muscular contractions of the uterus during pregnancy; intended to expel the fetus
  There are three phases of labor:
    —first stage begins with contractions and ends with the full dilation of the cervix
    —second stage begins with the full dilation of the cervix and ends with the delivery of the infant
    —third stage begins with the delivery of the infant and ends with the delivery of the placenta

- the secretion of milk

- an abnormality in a body part due to injury or disease

leukemia

limb presentation

liver

MEDICAL / OBSTETRICS / GYNECOLOGY

- a disease of the blood, characterized by excessive production of white blood cells

- occurrence during childbirth in which the infant's leg or arm is the presenting part during delivery

- a bodily organ located in the right upper quadrant of the abdomen that detoxifies drugs, secretes bile, and produces glucose

lymphatic system

malignant

meconium

- the body system responsible for maintaining the internal fluid system of the body

- cancerous; likely to become worse and result in death

- fetal stool

meconium stain

melena

meninges

- fecal contamination of amniotic fluid, giving off a green or brownish color and often indicating complications of birth and fetal distress

- stool containing blood, with a black, tarry appearance

- three layers of brain and spinal-cord covering: the dura mater (outermost), the arachnoid (middle), and the pia mater (innermost)

meningitis

menstruation

metabolism

- inflammation of the meninges

- the periodic discharge and shedding of the uterine lining in females

- the biochemical reactions that take place in the body, to provide energy and growth, and to support other bodily functions

miosis

miscarriage

motor division

- excessive constriction of the pupil in the eye

- the spontaneous loss of an embryo or fetus prior to the twentieth week of pregnancy

- division of the peripheral nervous system that transmits impulses to muscles and glands

mucous membrane

mucus

multigravida

MEDICAL / OBSTETRICS / GYNECOLOGY

- membranes containing mucous-producing glands that line and protect various organs

- slippery secretion that serves to lubricate and protect various bodily surfaces

- having experienced more than one pregnancy

mydriasis

nausea

necrosis

- prolonged dilation of the pupil in the eye

- the sensation resulting from stomach illness, typically prior to vomiting

- death of bodily tissue

nephritis

nephron

nervous system

- acute or chronic inflammation of the kidney

- the unit of the kidney that performs the actual filtration of blood

- the bodily system consisting of the brain, spinal cord, and nerves

neuralgia

neurogenic shock

nystagmus

- pain in one or more of the nerves in the body

- hypoperfusion due to nervous system dysfunction, resulting in dilation of blood vessels

- an involuntary rhythmic jerking of the eyeball; sometimes a sign of toxicity

ocular

oliguria

ophthalmoscope

- related to the eye

- minimal urine output

- an instrument used to examine the inside of the eye

organophosphates

orthostatic hypotension

osteoporosis

- a category of toxic chemicals that are used as pesticides and as dangerous weapons

- low blood pressure, usually transient, as one changes from a sitting to a standing position

- decrease in bone density, causing an increased likelihood of a bone break

otoscope

ovary

ovulation

- instrument used to examine the inside of the ear and nose

- the female sex organ in which eggs and female hormones are produced

- process whereby an ovum, or egg cell, is released

pallor

palsy

pancreas

MEDICAL / OBSTETRICS / GYNECOLOGY

- very pale skin

- paralysis

- an organ of the digestive system that secretes digestive enzymes

pancreatitis

paralysis

paranoia

- inflammation of the pancreas

- loss of the ability to move a body part

- abnormal or unrealistic suspiciousness, typically with exaggerated feelings of persecution

parasympathetic nervous system

paresis

paresthesia

- part of the autonomic nervous system that controls vegetative functions of the body, such as digestion; works in conjunction with the sympathetic nervous system to keep the body in balance

- weakness or slight paralysis

- a sensation of numbness or tingling

paroxysmal

pathogen

pathological

- symptoms occurring suddenly and usually intensely

- an organism that causes infection

- diseased

pedal

peptic

perineum

- pertaining to the foot

- pertaining to digestion

- area between the anus and the external genitalia

peripheral nervous system (PNS)

peristalsis

peritoneal cavity

- the nerves that connect the body and its organs to the central nervous system; is broken into motor and sensory divisions

- the muscular contractions of the intestines that move food along during digestion

- abdominal cavity

peritoneum

peritonitis

petit mal seizure

- the membrane that surrounds the abdominal cavity and consists of two layers: the visceral, which surrounds the organs; and the parietal, which lines the abdominal cavity

- inflammation of the peritoneum

- an absence or momentary loss of awareness without muscle jerking or other motor dysfunction

phlebitis

phobia

photophobia

MEDICAL / OBSTETRICS / GYNECOLOGY

- inflammation of a vein

- a persistent, irrational fear

- sensitivity to light

[352]

pia mater

placenta

placenta previa

- the innermost layer of the meninges, covering the brain

- the afterbirth; an organ attached to the uterine wall and connected to the fetus, which mediates metabolic exchange

- condition in which the placenta is attached very low in the uterus and potentially over the cervical opening; a normal vaginal delivery is not possible in this case

polydipsia

polyphagia

polyuria

- excessive thirst

- excessive hunger

- excessive urination

postictal

preeclampsia

primigravida

MEDICAL / OBSTETRICS / GYNECOLOGY

- the period of decreased consciousness that occurs after a grand mal seizure

- a pregnancy complication that is typically characterized by high blood pressure, as well as indications of organ system damage (often to the kidneys)

- a term that refers to a woman who is pregnant for the first time

prolapsed cord

psychosis

psychotic

- an urgent situation during childbirth that occurs when the umbilical cord is protruding from the vagina, causing the infant's head to compress the cord against the vaginal wall

- major psychological disorder, in which a patient is unable to discern reality

- an individual with a psychosis

referred pain

reflex

renal

- pain felt somewhere other than the injured or diseased part of the body

- involuntary reaction to a stimulus

- pertaining to the kidney

retroperitoneum

seizure

sensory division

- the area behind the peritoneum, where the kidneys and pancreas are located

- a discharge of electrical activity in the brain, causing some type of neurological dysfunction—from a mild period of unresponsiveness to a full-body, uncontrollable contraction of a muscle group

- the part of the peripheral nervous system that transmits sensory information to the central nervous system

sepsis

sickle cell anemia

somatic nervous system

- infection

- chronic anemia, characterized by sickle- or crescent-shaped red blood cells and destruction of red blood cells

- the part of the nervous system that transmits voluntary impulses to the muscles and organs of the body

spasm

spontaneous abortion

status asthmaticus

- a sudden involuntary contraction of a muscle or constriction of a passageway

- miscarriage; delivery of the fetus and placenta prior to the twentieth week of pregnancy

- a severe asthma attack that is not stopped by epinephrine or bronchodilator administration

status epilepticus

stillborn

stroke

- repeated seizures or seizure activity without a period of consciousness

- born dead and unable to be resuscitated

- a brain attack or cerebrovascular accident (CVA); damage of a portion of the brain due to lack of blood flow

sudden infant death syndrome (SIDS)

sympathetic nervous system

syncope

- the abrupt and unexplained death of a child younger than the age of one year

- part of the autonomic nervous system that readies the body to react to stressful situations; works in conjunction with parasympathetic nervous system to maintain balance

- temporary loss of consciousness; fainting

testes

tetanus

tetany

- sperm-producing genitalia, located in the scrotum

- a bacterial infection that causes muscle spasms of the jaw and clenched teeth (lockjaw)

- involuntary muscle twitching or spasms, typically due to calcium imbalance

therapeutic abortion

threatened abortion

tinnitus

- an induced termination of pregnancy, to protect the health of the mother

- vaginal bleeding, indicating the possibility or threat of a spontaneous miscarriage

- ringing or buzzing noise in the ears, sometimes the result of drug toxicity

toxemia

toxin

transient ischemic attack (TIA)

- the presence of a toxic substance in the blood

- poison from a plant, animal, or bacteria

- a ministroke or neurological event with temporary symptoms lasting less than 24 hours

transverse lie

tremor

trimester

MEDICAL / OBSTETRICS / GYNECOLOGY

- an abnormal fetal presentation where the baby is sideways in the uterus

- an involuntary twitching or fine movement, usually in the hands

- a period of three months, usually in reference to the three trimesters of pregnancy

trismus

ulcer

umbilical cord

- a jaw muscle spasm causing clenched teeth

- open, craterlike sore on the skin or mucous membrane

- the cord containing blood vessels (one vein and two arteries) that connects the fetus to the placenta

umbilicus

urea

urinary retention

- the navel

- a waste product of the body that contains nitrogen

- the inability to urinate

urine

urticaria

uterus

- fluid waste secreted by the kidneys and stored in the urinary bladder

- hives

- womb; the pear-shaped internal female reproductive organ

vagina

venereal disease

vertex presentation

- the birth canal

- a sexually transmitted, contagious disease

- the normal position of the fetus during delivery, with the head first

vertigo

vulva

- physical and mental dizziness and/or sensation of confusion

- external female genitalia

a-

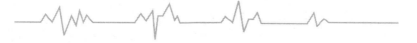

abandonment

abduction

- a prefix meaning *without* or *lack of*

- leaving a patient after care has begun, and prior to handing care over to someone of equal or greater medical training, without giving a patient sufficient time to find another suitable provider

- movement away from the midline of the body

adduction

adrenergic

advanced directive

- movement toward the midline of the body

- 1. related to sympathetic nerve fibers of the autonomic nervous system; 2. related to the adrenal gland, where epinephrine and norepinephrine are made

- a document that expresses a patient's wishes in reference to future medical care, including do not resuscitate orders, living wills, and organ donation

advanced life support (ALS)

albuterol

anterior

EMS OPERATIONS

- treatment that involves medications and procedures that could have serious side effects or complications; most ALS is provided by a paramedic or AEMT, but some may be provided by an EMT

- a bronchodilator/beta 2 agonist medication

- the front surface of a body or body part

atrophy

auto-injector

basic life support (BLS)

- a decrease in cell size due to nerve damage, malnutrition, or a decrease in workload

- a type of preloaded medication syringe with spring-loaded action that makes injecting quick and easy, especially for self-administration

- the use of basic, noninvasive techniques to sustain life or stabilize ill or injured persons

bilateral

blood pressure

brady-

- both sides

- the pressure (measured in millimeters of mercury, mmHg) of the blood against the blood vessel wall; systolic pressure is measured after the heart contracts (contraction); diastolic pressure is measured before the heart contracts (relaxation)

- a prefix meaning *slow*

CHART

CHEATED

chemical name

EMS OPERATIONS

- An acronym for the format of a patient care narrative:
    - **C**—Chief complaint
    - **H**—History of present illness and patient's past history
    - **A**—Assessment, including primary, secondary, and ongoing assessments
    - **R**—Rx/treatment rendered to the patient
    - **T**—Transport via, to where, and any changes during transport

- An acronym for the format of a patient care narrative:
    - **C**—Chief complaint
    - **H**—History of the present illness and patient's past history
    - **E**—Exam, including the primary and secondary survey
    - **A**—Assessment or your impression of the patient's condition
    - **T**—Treatment rendered to the patient
    - **E**—Evaluation of the treatments and ongoing evaluation
    - **D**—Disposition of the patient

- name of a drug that describes its chemical makeup

chief complaint

cold zone

contraindication

EMS OPERATIONS

- the primary reason why a patient has sought medical care

- the uncontaminated safe area at the scene of a hazardous materials incident; this is where the command post and support functions are usually located

- a signal that indicates when not to do a specific procedure or give a medication

critical incident stress debriefing (CISD)

critical incident stress defusing

critical incident stress management (CISM)

- a formal discussion session involving EMS personnel who participated in an emotionally challenging event; it is usually held 24 to 72 hours after the event

- an informal meeting to help responders with expectations of what they might experience after a stressful incident; it may occur at the scene of the incident or shortly after

- methods used to assist emergency personnel in coping with stressful calls, such as line of duty deaths or injuries to children

EMS OPERATIONS

decontamination

Do Not Resuscitate order (DNR)

dys-

- the removal of dangerous chemicals or infectious agents

- a written order, completed by a patient, a patient's legal representative, or a physician, indicating a patient's wishes in the event that he or she experiences cardiopulmonary arrest

- a prefix meaning *difficult* or *painful*

-ectomy

-emia

epi-

- a suffix meaning *surgical removal*

- a suffix meaning *blood*

- a prefix meaning *over* or *upon*

extricate

flammable

Fowler's position

- to free from entrapment

- capable of being easily ignited

- a standard, semi-sitting patient position

gastro-

generic name

geriatric

- a word root referring to the stomach

- name of a drug that is nonproprietary, identifing the chemical in the drug; is not capitalized

- pertaining to the elderly

Good Samaritan laws

hem-

hemat-

EMS OPERATIONS

- laws designed to protect individuals who stop to render aid at the scene of an accident; these laws minimize the liability of someone acting to the best of his or her abilities and training

- a word root meaning *blood*

- a word root meaning *blood*

hemi-

HEPA mask

hepat-

EMS OPERATIONS

- a prefix meaning *half*

- a high-efficiency particulate air filter that blocks microparticles and prevents transmission of airborne communicable disease

- a word root meaning *liver*

hot zone

hyper-

hypo-

- the area at an incident where a direct threat exists, requiring specific training or personal protective equipment to enter; usually used during a hazardous materials incident

- a prefix meaning *too much*

- a prefix meaning *too little*

implied consent

incident command system (ICS)

indication

- the principle of consent that assumes a severely ill, unconscious person would want medical intervention if he or she were able to consent

- a management system that coordinates emergency response and operations involving multiple personnel or jurisdictions

- a signal that it is appropriate to use a certain medication or procedure

inferior

informed consent

injection

- away from the head and toward the feet

- permission or agreement to medical treatment and/or transport based upon receipt of appropriate information

- a route of medication administration or exposure to a toxin where the agent is introduce under the skin (subcutaneous) or into a muscle (intramuscular), vein (intravenous), or bone (intraosseous)

innocuous

insufficiency

intramuscular

EMS OPERATIONS

- not harmful

- inadequacy

- into the muscle

intraosseous

intravenous (IV)

involuntary consent

- into the bone; an alternate route for fluids and medications for patients when intravenous access is not available

- into a vein

- treatment or transportation against one's will, usually mandated by a court or statute

-itis

kinematics

lateral

- a suffix meaning *inflammation*

- the study of motion and energy

- an anatomical term indicating a position away from the middle of the body

lateral recumbent position

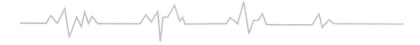

liability

living will

- posture assumed by placing a patient on his or her side

- the state of being legally responsible or susceptible

- a legal document containing specific instructions regarding express medical decisions should one become incompetent; often intended to prevent resuscitative efforts or mechanical support

log rolling

medial

morbidity

- a procedure to move a patient while keeping the head and spine aligned

- toward the midline or middle

- degree or severity of an illness

mortality

multiple casualty incident (MCI)

narcotic

- rate of death in a population

- a disaster or incident where there are multiple injured or ill victims

- a drug, an opiod, often used to produce euphoria and relaxation; its antagonist is naloxone

nature of illness

negligence

nephr-

- a general description of the medical condition that is causing the illness requiring an EMS response

- failure to provide a standard of care that a reasonable and similarly trained person would provide
    Four principles must be proven for negligence to have occurred:
        1. a duty to act must be present
        2. this duty must be violated
        3. there must be an injury
        4. the injury must have been caused by the failure to act

- a word root meaning *kidney*

neuroleptics

nitroglycerin

normal saline (ns)

- a category of drugs used to manage psychosis; antipsychotics

- a medication to dilate coronary arteries during episodes of coronary distress

- a 0.9 percent salt (sodium chloride) solution that is similar to body fluid; it can be administered in an intravenous solution or used as an irrigating solution on a wound

offline medical direction

online medical direction

percutaneous

EMS OPERATIONS

- indirect medical direction, including protocols and written orders; system oversight that occurs before and after an EMS call

- direct medical direction that includes voice communication between EMS personnel and a physician

- performed through the skin

peri-

peripheral

personal protective equipment (PPE)

- a prefix meaning *around*

- anatomical term indicating distance away from the center; relating to the peripheral nervous system

- protection from communicable diseases or hazardous materials with eyewear, gloves, gown, mask, helmet, or other protective wear

pharmacokinetics

poly-

posterior

- the study of the absorption, distribution, metabolism, and excretion of drugs in the body

- a prefix meaning *excessive*

- back side of the body or of an organ

potentiation

proximal

quadrant

- an enhanced effect of a drug caused by the simultaneous use of another drug

- an anatomical term meaning closer to the body on an extremity; opposite of distal

- placing an imaginary line through the umbilicus both sagittally and transversely, therefore dividing the abdomen into four sections: upper right quadrant (URQ); upper left quadrant (ULQ); lower right quadrant (LRQ); and lower left quadrant (LLQ)

radial

reasonable force

recovery position

- pertaining to the wrist

- appropriate force to restrain or subdue an individual when necessary

- positioning an individual on his or her left side (left lateral recumbent) to allow secretions to drain out of the mouth; used to assist in airway maintenance in a breathing but unresponsive patient without trauma

-rrhage

saline

scope of practice

- a suffix meaning *excessive flow*

- salt solution

- the specified practices and procedures allowed for a specific healthcare provider, usually determined by state statute

sedative

side effect

SOAP

- a category of medication that depresses the central nervous system, causing sedation and/or sleep

- an undesired effect of a drug

- An acronym for the format of a patient care narrative:
    - **S**—Subjective, or information you hear (symptoms, chief complaint, history)
    - **O**—Objective, or information you see or feel (examination findings)
    - **A**—Assessment: your impression of the patient's condition
    - **P**—Plan you develop for the care and transport of the patient

sphygmomanometer

standard of care

standard precautions (BSI)

- a blood pressure cuff

- the minimal level of appropriate care or performance criteria provided in a particular community

- formerly known as Body Substance Isolation (BSI); the practice of isolating all body fluids or substances to reduce the risk of possible infection

stasis

steroid

stimulant

- slowing or sluggishness of the flow of a liquid, often blood or urine

- a category of medication with a 17-carbon, four-ring arrangement

- a category of drug that stimulates the central nervous system and increases body activity

sub-

subcutaneous

subdiaphragmatic

EMS OPERATIONS

- a prefix meaning *under*

- the tissue beneath the skin

- below the diaphragm

sublingual

superior

supine

- under the tongue

- a directional anatomy term, meaning toward the top or the head

- lying on the back, faceup

supraclavicular

sympatholytic

sympathomimetic

- above the clavicle

- antiadrenergic; a drug that blocks the action of the sympathetic nervous system

- a drug that mimics the action of the sympathetic nervous system

synergism

systemic

therapeutic action

- the combination of two drugs, where the result is greater than the sum of each drug individually

- pertaining to the entire body system

- the desired effect of a drug

thrombolytic

tolerance

toxic

- a category of drugs that break down or dissolve thrombi, destroying clots

- diminished effect of a drug due to repeated use, often requiring an increase in dosage to achieve the same effect

- poisonous

trade name

Trendelenburg position

triage

EMS OPERATIONS

- brand name or manufacturer's name of a medication

- position where a patient's feet and legs are elevated higher than the head; used during hypovolemic shock

- the sorting of patients based on priority of medical care
    There are two levels of triage:
    —Primary occurs where the patients are injured and follows the START and JumpSTART triage systems
    —Secondary usually occurs in the treatment area and takes into account a brief patient assessment and vital signs

unilateral

universal precautions

uppers

- occurring on one side of the body

- concept of infection control that assumes every patient is carrying a potential infection; gloves, mask, and protective eyewear are used when blood or body secretions are contacted; now referred to as standard precautions

- slang for a category of drugs that stimulate the central nervous system

vas-

venipuncture

venom

- a word root meaning *vessel*

- the puncture of a vein, usually for the purpose of obtaining a blood sample or starting an intravenous infusion

- toxic fluid secreted by some animals and insects

venous access device (VAD)

viable

visceral

- a surgically implanted device that allows continuous access to veins

- potential to survive or live

- internal tissues and organs

vital signs

warm zone

- an individual's pulse and respiratory rate, blood pressure, temperature, and skin color

- the area at an incident where responders may be exposed to a hazard/threat from the hot zone and specialized training and equipment may be required to support hot zone operations, but not enter the hot zone; in a HazMat incident, the warm zone is where decontamination is established

APPENDIX A:

AIRWAY OBSTRUCTION PROCEDURES

Conscious Patient (Adult):

Can the patient speak?

➤ YES—partial airway obstruction; support with O2

➤ NO—complete obstruction; perform Heimlich maneuver

- Ask the patient if you can help
- Position yourself behind the patient
- Form a fist with thumb tucked in
- Support your fist with the other hand
- Place your fist midway between the naval and xiphoid process
- Thrust up and back
- Continue thrusts until the object is expelled or the patient loses consciousness

Conscious Patient (Child Aged 1–8 Years):

Same procedure as above, only using force appropriate for the patient's size

Conscious Pregnant or Obese Patient:

Same as conscious patient, but place your hands in the middle of the sternum

Conscious Infant:

➤ Place the patient prone on your arm with the legs straddling your arm

➤ Hold the patient's head in your hand

➤ Hold the patient head-down to assist with expelling the obstruction
➤ Administer five (5) back blows with the palm of your hand
➤ Sandwich the patient between your arms and turn the patient supine, still supporting his or her head
➤ Administer five (5) chest thrusts using the same technique as chest compressions
➤ Check the airway for the obstruction; if seen, remove it
➤ Attempt ventilations
➤ If unsuccessful, readjust the airway and attempt to ventilate
➤ If still unsuccessful, repeat the steps until the object is expelled or the patient loses consciousness

Unconscious patients:
➤ Open the airway and attempt to visualize the obstruction
➤ If seen, remove the obstruction and attempt to ventilate
➤ If nothing is seen in the airway, attempt ventilations and proceed to CPR appropriate for the age of the patient

APPENDIX B:

APGAR SCORE

Eval/Score	0	1	2
Appearance	Central cyanosis	Pink body, mild cyanosis of extremities	Entire body is pink
Pulse	None	< 100	≥100
Grimace	No reaction to stimuli	Weak cry with little or no reaction to stimuli	Strong cry and reaction to stimuli
Activity	Limp with no muscle tone	Weak resistance to leg straightening	Strong resistance to straightening of legs/hips
Respirations	None	Slow or irregular	Adequate

APPENDIX C:
AXIAL AND APPENDICULAR SKELETON

AXIAL SKELETON

APPENDICULAR SKELETON

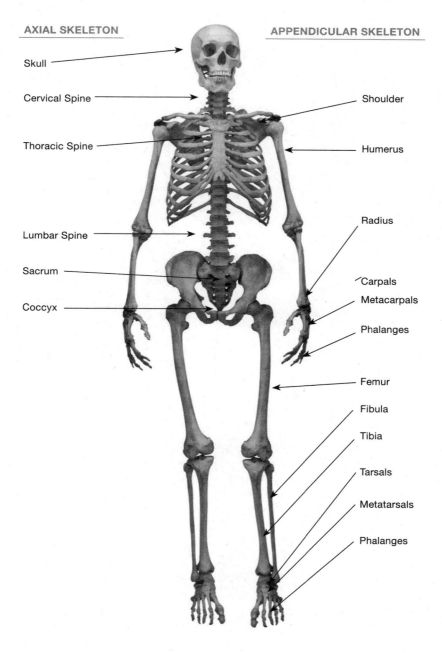

Skull

Cervical Spine

Thoracic Spine

Lumbar Spine

Sacrum

Coccyx

Shoulder

Humerus

Radius

Carpals

Metacarpals

Phalanges

Femur

Fibula

Tibia

Tarsals

Metatarsals

Phalanges

APPENDIX D:

THE THORAX AND MEDIASTINUM

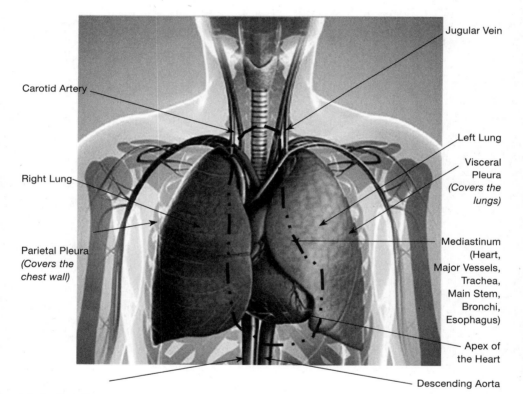

Jugular Vein

Carotid Artery

Left Lung

Visceral
Pleura
(Covers the
lungs)

Right Lung

Parietal Pleura
(Covers the
chest wall)

Mediastinum
(Heart,
Major Vessels,
Trachea,
Main Stem,
Bronchi,
Esophagus)

Apex of
the Heart

Descending Aorta

Inferior Vena Cava

APPENDIX E:

THE HEART

HEART ANATOMY

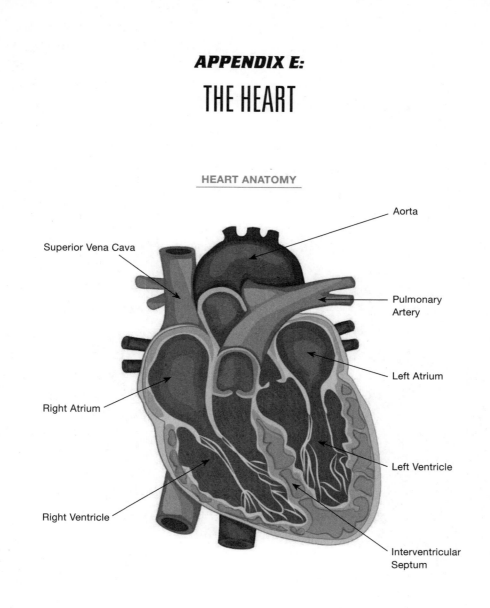

Aorta

Superior Vena Cava

Pulmonary Artery

Left Atrium

Right Atrium

Left Ventricle

Right Ventricle

Interventricular Septum

APPENDIX F:

NORMAL CONDUCTION OF THE HEART

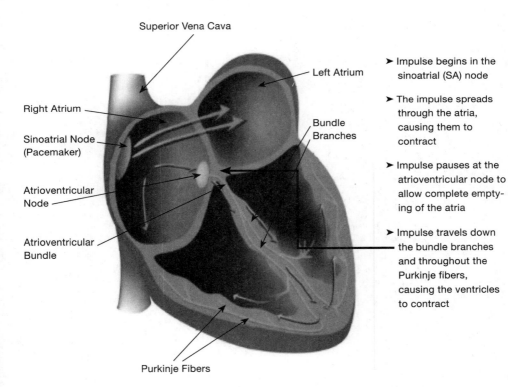

Superior Vena Cava

Left Atrium

Right Atrium

Sinoatrial Node
(Pacemaker)

Atrioventricular
Node

Atrioventricular
Bundle

Bundle
Branches

Purkinje Fibers

➤ Impulse begins in the
sinoatrial (SA) node

➤ The impulse spreads
through the atria,
causing them to
contract

➤ Impulse pauses at the
atrioventricular node to
allow complete empty-
ing of the atria

➤ Impulse travels down
the bundle branches
and throughout the
Purkinje fibers,
causing the ventricles
to contract

APPENDIX G:

GLASGOW COMA SCALE

GLASGOW COMA SCORE		
Eye Opening Response		**Score**
Spontaneous	4	
To verbal stimuli	3	
To painful stimuli	2	
No response	1	
Verbal Response		
Oriented to name, place, time, and event	5	
Confused statements	4	
Inappropriate words	3	
Incomprehensible sounds	2	
No response	1	
Motor Response		
Obeys commands	6	
Localizes pain	5	
Withdraws from pain	4	
Abnormal flexion to pain (decorticate posturing)	3	
Abnormal extension (decerebrate posturing)	2	
No response	1	
Total		

The GCS can add up to between 15 and 3, with decreasing scores indicating an increase in the severity of injury. A GCS of 13 or less indicates a need for rapid transport and short scene time, and a GCS of 8 indicates a serious brain injury requiring transport to a Level I Trauma Center.

APPENDIX H:

REVISED TRAUMA SCORE

REVISED TRAUMA SCORE		
GCS Score		**Score**
13–15	4	
9–12	3	
6–8	2	
4–5	1	
3	0	
Systolic Blood Pressure		
> 89	4	
76–89	3	
50–75	2	
1–49	1	
0	0	
Respiratory Rate		
10–29	4	
> 29	3	
6–9	2	
1–5	1	
0	0	
Total		

The RTS is another valuable scoring system in determining the probability of survival; the EMT sets the baseline by obtaining an initial RTS.

APPENDIX I:

RULE OF NINES

INFANT

Entire head	= 18%
Anterior torso	= 18%
Posterior torso	= 18%
Each arm	= 9%
Each leg	= 13.5%
Genitalia	= 1%
Total	= 100%

CHILD:

Varies with age and textbook.

ADULT:

Head	= 9%
Anterior torso	= 18%
Posterior torso	= 18%
Each arm	= 9%
Each leg	= 18%
Genitalia	= 1%
Total	= 100%

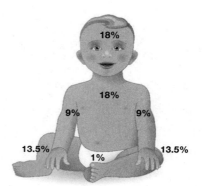

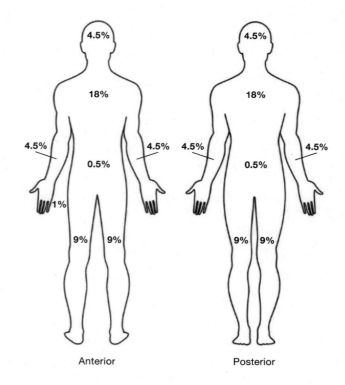

Anterior   Posterior

APPENDIX J:

START TRIAGE

1. All patients that can walk are tagged **GREEN** and directed to the treatment area

2. Assess the nonambulatory patients for respiratory effort
   a. If none, open the airway
      i. No spontaneous respirations, tag them **DECEASED**
      ii. Spontaneous respirations, tag them **RED**
   b. If they have spontaneous respirations, assess the rate
      i. > 30 per minute, tag them **RED**
      ii. < 30 per minute, move to the next assessment

3. Assess the radial pulse or capillary refill
   a. If no pulse or capillary refill is > 2 seconds, tag them **RED**
   b. If the radial pulse is present or capillary refill is < 2 seconds, move to the next step

4. Assess the patient's mental status
   a. If they cannot obey simple commands, tag them **RED**
   b. If they can obey simple commands, tag them **YELLOW**

JUMPSTART TRIAGE

- All children too young to walk shall be moved to the treatment area immediately for secondary triage and treatment
- All children old enough to walk and can are tagged **GREEN** and directed to the treatment area
- Assess the nonambulatory children for respiratory effort
- If none, open the airway
- No spontaneous respirations, check for a pulse
- No pulse, tag them **DECEASED**
- Radial/brachial pulse present, give 5 rescue breaths
- No spontaneous respirations, tag them **DECEASED**
- Spontaneous respirations, tag them **RED**
- Assess rate of spontaneous respirations
- < 15 or > 45, tag **RED**
- > 15 or < 45, move to the next assessment
- Assess the radial pulse or capillary refill
- No pulse or capillary refill > 2 seconds, tag **RED**
- Pulse is present or capillary refill < 2 seconds, move to the next assessment
- Assess mental status using AVPU
- Inappropriate response to pain (decerebrate/decorticate posturing) or unresponsive, tag **RED**
- Appropriate response to pain (localize/withdraw), responds to verbal, or alert, tag **YELLOW**